LOW HISTAMINE COOKBOOK

Delicious Easy-to-Follow Recipes and Meal Plans for Managing Histamine Intolerance.

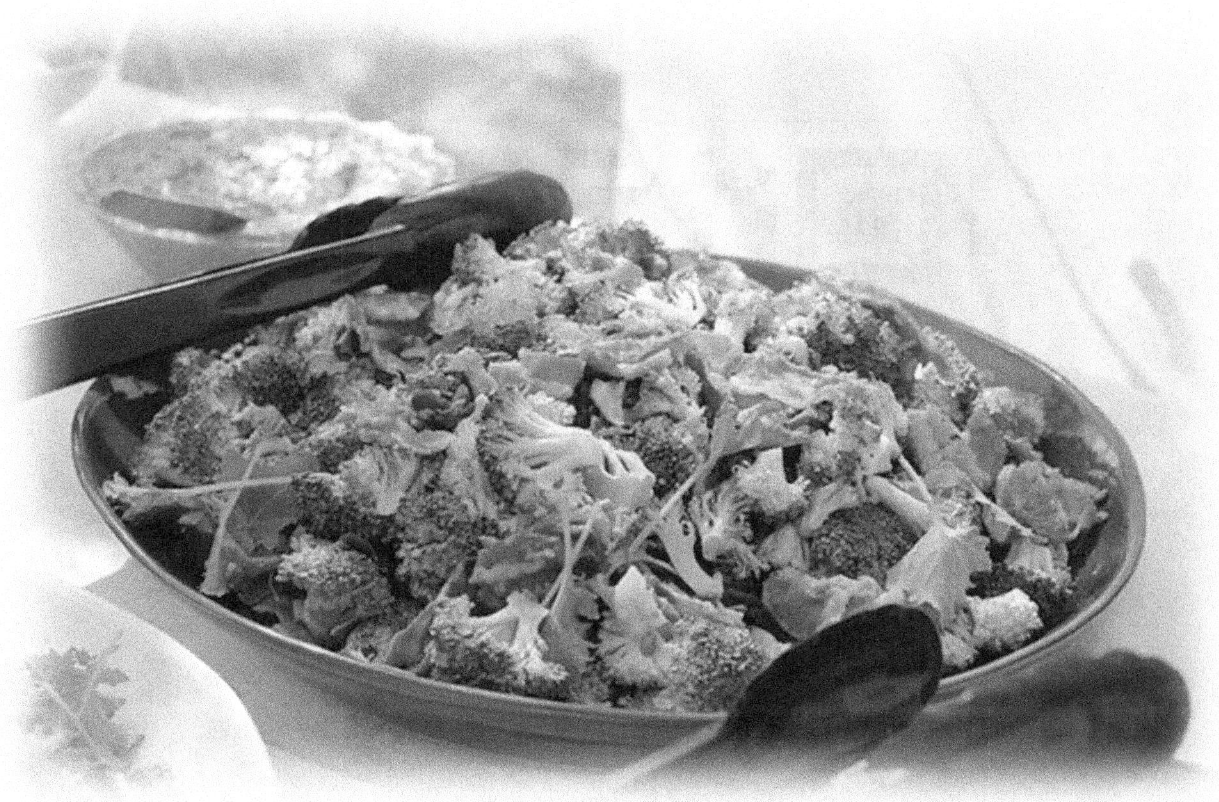

CHRISTIANA WHITE

GAIN ACCESS TO MORE BOOKS

DISCLAIMER

The recipes in this cookbook are provided for informational purposes only and are not intended as medical or professional advice. While the author and publisher have made every effort to ensure the accuracy and effectiveness of the recipes, they are not responsible for any adverse effects r consequences resulting from the use of the suggestions herein.

The information in this cookbook should not replace professional advice. Readers are advised to consult a healthcare provider or a culinary professional before making any significant changes to their diet or cooking practices.

Nutritional information is approximate and should be used as a guide only. Variations may occur due to product availability, food preparation, portion size, and other factors.

The author and publisher disclaim any liability in connection with the use of this information. It is the reader's responsibility to determine the value and quality of any recipe or instructions provided for food preparation and to determine the nutritional adequacy of the food to be consumed.

ABOUT THE AUTHOR

When it comes to tasty and nutritious cookbooks that turn wellness into a delightful journey, Christiana White is the author you turn to. She approaches cooking from a new angle and has a passion for creating wholesome food.

Motivated by her own pursuit of health, Christiana's books on Amazon are brimming with delectable recipes that demonstrate that eating healthily can be both simple and enjoyable. Her creative method makes cooking approachable to all skill levels by fusing entire, simple foods with flavors from around the world.

Readers of Christiana's meals gush about the beneficial effects her foods have on their lives outside of the kitchen. Her books are more than just recipes; they're guides for a happier, better way of life, resulting in everything from more energy to a revitalized passion for cooking.

Come along with Christiana to discover how to turn your meals into satisfying and joyful experiences. Discover the delightful intersection of health and flavor by delving into the colourful world of her cookbooks.

TABLE OF CONTENTS.

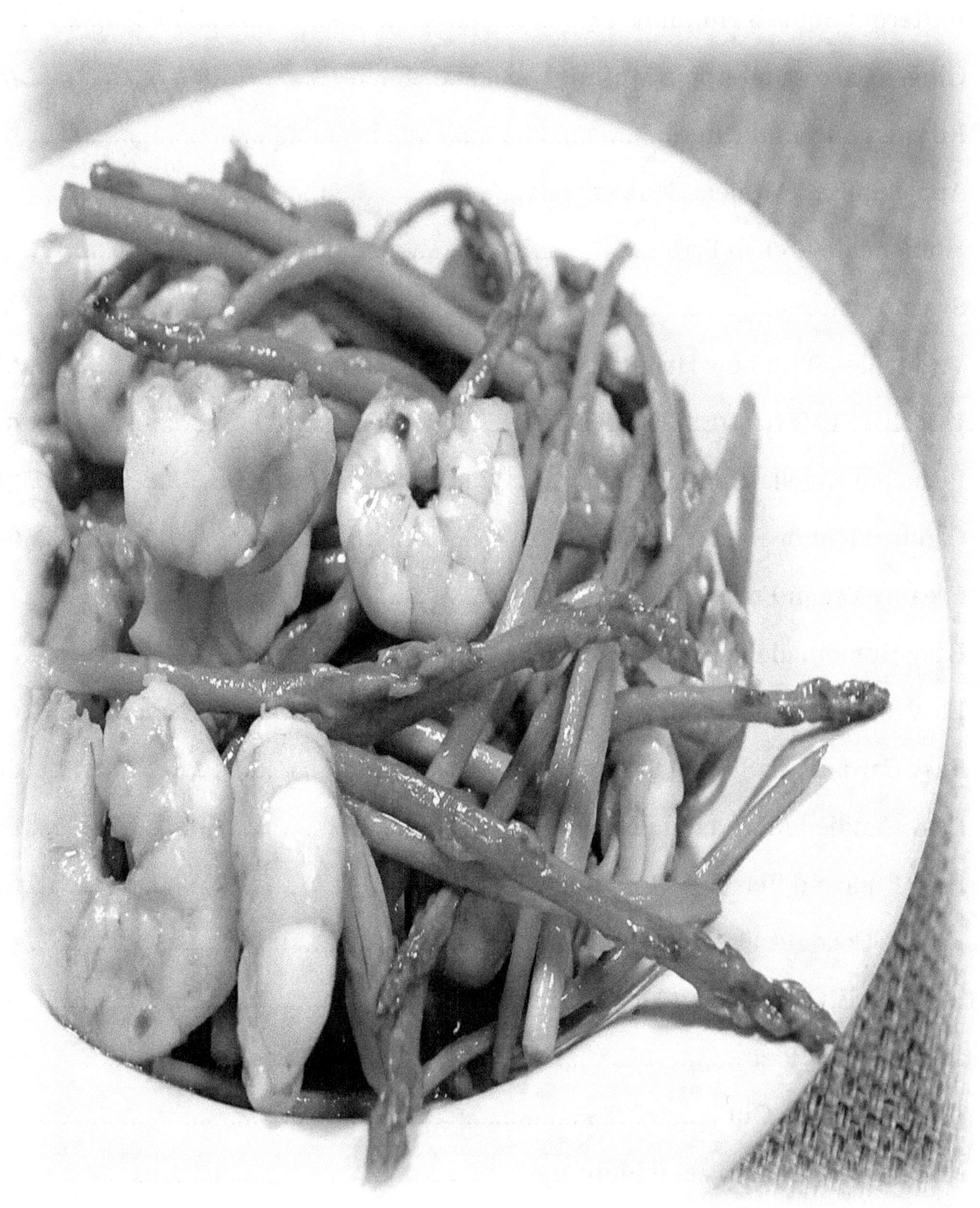

INTRODUCTION

Have you ever felt that your body is fighting a battle against the meals you enjoy? Unexpected symptoms may include rashes, headaches, and stomach issues. If this sounds similar, you aren't alone. Millions of people suffer with histamine intolerance, a condition in which the body struggles to break down histamine, a chemical contained in many everyday foods.

It might be difficult to navigate the culinary world when you have histamine sensitivity. It's stressful to miss out on wonderful meals and social occasions because you're constantly worried of sparking a reaction. But I am here to tell you that it does not have to be this way.

Imagine a life in which you may enjoy delectable meals without fear of histamine excess. A life in which you can boldly try new dishes and ingredients, knowing they won't make you unhappy. That is the promise of this cookbook.

These pages provide numerous tempting recipes that are both delicious and low in histamine. From hearty breakfasts to filling dinners, tasty snacks to delectable sweets, this cookbook has something for everyone. But it isn't only recipes. You'll discover important methods for dealing with histamine intolerance, navigating grocery shops, and dining out with confidence.

As someone who has personally walked this path, I understand the difficulties you confront. I've spent countless hours researching and experimenting with low-histamine cuisine, and I'm excited to share my insights and experiences with you.

This cookbook is your ticket to a world of culinary possibilities. It's an invitation to rediscover the joy of eating, nourish your body with healthy foods, and reclaim your health and well-being. Let us go on this amazing journey together!

CHAPTER ONE

The Science of Histamines

Histamine, a naturally occurring chemical in our bodies, is essential for immunological response, digestion, and brain function. However, for people who are histamine intolerant, this usually useful chemical might cause discomfort and anguish.

What is histamine?

Histamine is a chemical messenger that belongs to the group of chemicals known as biogenic amines. It is produced by numerous cells in the body, most notably mast cells and basophils, as part of the immune system's response to allergens, injuries, or infections.

How Does Histamine Work?

When the body detects a perceived threat, such as an allergen, mast cells release histamine into the bloodstream. Histamine then attaches to certain receptors (H1, H2, H3, and H4) on various cells throughout the body, causing a series of events.

These reactions can result in a variety of symptoms, including:

- Skin symptoms: itching, hives, flushing
- Respiratory system symptoms: sneezing, runny nose, congestion, asthma.
- Digestive symptoms include nausea, vomiting, diarrhea, and abdominal pain.
- Cardiovascular system: rapid heartbeat and low blood pressure.
- Nervous system: headaches, dizziness, and anxiety.

Understand Histamine Intolerance

Histamine intolerance occurs when histamine levels exceed the body's ability to break them down. Several things can contribute to this, including:

- Reduced DAO Enzyme Activity: Diamine oxidase (DAO) is the principal enzyme that degrades ingested histamine. Individuals with histamine intolerance frequently have diminished DAO activity, resulting in a buildup of histamine in the body.
- Increased Histamine Production: Certain foods and environmental factors can cause mast cells to release an excessive quantity of histamine.
- Impaired Histamine. Metabolism: Genetic differences or some drugs can impair the body's capacity to metabolize histamine efficiently.

The low-histamine diet seeks to minimize the body's total histamine burden by avoiding or restricting high-histamine foods while emphasizing foods that are low in histamine and/or assist histamine breakdown. Individuals with histamine intolerance may benefit from this method in terms of symptom relief and improved quality of life.

While avoiding high-histamine meals is critical for controlling histamine sensitivity, it's also necessary to focus on:

- Nutrient-Dense Foods: Eat whole, unprocessed foods high in nutrients, vitamins, and minerals to promote general health and well-being.
- Gut Health: A healthy gut microbiota helps regulate histamine levels. Probiotics and prebiotics can help maintain a healthy gut environment.
- Stress Management: Chronic stress might worsen histamine intolerance symptoms. Finding appropriate stress-management techniques, such as yoga, meditation, or spending time outside, might be therapeutic.

This cookbook aims to provide you with the knowledge and tools you need to flourish on a low-histamine diet. You may regain control of your health and well-being by learning about histamine science and making informed food choices.

The Benefits of a Low Histamine Diet

For many who suffer from histamine intolerance, starting a reduced histamine diet can be a life-changing event. By adopting conscious eating choices and understanding the complexities of histamine metabolism, you can gain a wealth of benefits in addition to symptom relief.

Reduced Or Eliminated Symptoms.

The most immediate and important advantage of a reduced histamine diet is that it reduces or even eliminates histamine intolerance symptoms. By avoiding or restricting high-histamine meals and focusing on those that promote histamine breakdown, you can enjoy relief from:

- Digestive symptoms include nausea, vomiting, diarrhea, stomach pain, bloating, and acid reflux.
- Skin issues include itching, hives, eczema, and flushing.
- Respiratory issues: runny nose, congestion, sneezing, and asthma.
- Headaches and Migraines: Histamine is known to cause headaches and migraines. A low-histamine diet can considerably minimize their occurrence and severity.
- Weariness and Brain Fog: A histamine imbalance can lead to weariness, brain fog, and difficulties concentrating. A reduced histamine diet might boost mental clarity and energy levels.

Improved Gut Health

The gut microbiome plays an important role in histamine regulation. A low histamine diet frequently emphasizes complete, unprocessed foods, which can maintain a healthy gut microbiota. This can lead to:

- Improved Digestion: Proper gut flora can improve digestion and nutrient absorption, resulting in decreased bloating, gas, and pain.
- Stronger Immune System: A healthy stomach is critical for a strong immune system. You may boost your body's immune system by promoting a healthy microbiome.
- Reduced Inflammation: A healthy gut microbiome can help lower systemic inflammation, which is linked to a variety of chronic illnesses.

Enhanced Overall Well-being

A low histamine diet can have a tremendous impact on your general well-being.

- Increased Energy: Avoiding meals that cause histamine release and promoting effective histamine breakdown will help you feel more energized and vibrant.
- Improved Mood: Studies indicate a link between gut health and mental wellness. A low-histamine diet can help alleviate anxiety, melancholy, and mood changes.
- Improved Sleep: Histamine intolerance can interrupt sleeping habits. A reduced histamine diet can lead to deeper, more peaceful sleep.
- Improved Focus and Concentration: By minimizing brain fog and weariness, a reduced histamine diet helps boost cognitive performance and focus.

It's crucial to note that everyone's experience with histamine intolerance is different. While a low histamine diet can provide several benefits, it is critical to consult with a healthcare expert or certified dietitian to customize the diet to your unique needs and sensitivities.

Adopting a low histamine lifestyle will not only relieve symptoms, but also pave the way for better health, vitality, and a revitalized enthusiasm for life.

Detailed Food Lists: What To Enjoy and Avoid.

For people suffering from histamine intolerance, starting a reduced histamine diet can be a life-changing experience. To effectively manage symptoms, you must understand which meals to embrace and which to avoid.

Foods To Enjoy: These foods are generally considered low in histamine and are acceptable to incorporate into your diet:

- Fresh Meats & Poultry: Choose chilled, frozen, or fresh cuts of chicken, turkey, and other meats.
- Fresh/frozen fish: Look for histamine-free options such as hake, trout, and plaice.
- Eggs: Focus on the yolk, which contains less histamine.
- Fresh fruits are generally low in histamine, with the exception of strawberries, citrus, and avocados. Apples, pears, and peaches are terrific options.
- Fresh vegetables: Many are safe, such as artichokes, asparagus, broccoli, carrots, and potatoes. Avoid tomato, eggplant, and spinach.
- Grains: Rice, oats, millet, and gluten-free alternatives such as amaranth and quinoa are often well tolerated.
- Dairy Alternatives: Goat and sheep milk, as well as their products, can be suitable substitutes.
- Herbs and spices: While most fresh herbs are low in histamine, it's important to check for individual tolerance.

Foods to Avoid: These foods are known to be rich in histamine or can produce histamine in the body, and should generally be avoided:

- Aged and Fermented Foods: Examples include aged cheeses, fermented veggies, and meats such as salami and ham.
- Alcoholic beverages: Wine, beer, and champagne have high levels of histamine.
- Canned and processed foods: They frequently contain additional preservatives, which can raise histamine levels.
- Certain seafood: Canned fish and shellfish may have more histamine.
- Leftover Foods: Since histamine levels can rise over time, it's preferable to consume fresh.
- Certain fruits and vegetables: Citrus fruits, bananas, avocados, tomatoes, and spinach may be problematic.
- Avoid vinegar and vinegar-containing foods, such as ketchup, mayonnaise, and pickled items.
- Spices: Certain spices, such as chili powder and cinnamon, might cause histamine release.

Individual tolerance varies, so listen to your body and speak with a healthcare expert or dietician to adjust the diet to your personal needs. Keeping a food diary can be quite useful in determining which foods are best for you. By following these principles, you can develop a diet that promotes health and reduces histamine-related symptoms.

Creating a low histamine diet does not have to be costly or hard. With an emphasis on fresh, uncomplicated ingredients, you can create tasty meals that are both affordable and adhere to low histamine requirements. Here is a shopping list of must-have ingredients that are low in histamine, readily available, and reasonably priced:

Proteins:

- Freshly packaged or frozen chicken breasts, thighs, and drumsticks.
- Turkey (fresh cut or ground)
- Fresh or quickly thawed frozen fish (pollock, cod, trout, whitefish).

Dairy And Dairy Substitutes:

- Fresh milk (cow, goat, or sheep).
- Butter, unsalted
- Cream (to cook or whip)
- Cream cheese (mozzarella, cottage cheese, mascarpone, and ricotta).

Grains and Cereals:

- Potatoes (all types).
- Corn kernels (fresh or frozen).
- Rice (white, brown, and basmati)
- Oats (rolled or steel cut)
- Pasta, ordinary or gluten-free.
- Bakery items (freshly made bread and rolls).

Fruits and Vegetables:

- Apples.
- Peaches.
- Apricots.
- Melons (cantaloupe and honeydew)
- Mango.
- Persimmon
- Lychee.
- Cherries.
- Blackberries.
- Blueberries.
- Coconut (fresh, milk, and water)

Nuts and Seeds:

- Macadamias.
- Chestnuts.

Seasonings, Fats, And Oil:

- Olive oil (extra virgin).
- Coconut Oil
- Sunflower oil.
- Salt (Iodized or sea salt)
- Fresh herbs: parsley, cilantro, basil
- Garlic (fresh cloves).
- Ginger (fresh roots)

Sweets:

- Sugar (white, brown)
- Honey (preferably local and raw)

This list serves as a great foundation for your low histamine kitchen, allowing you to prepare a variety of dishes while staying within your budget. Remember to carefully verify the freshness and storage conditions of the ingredients, as histamine levels might rise with time.

Tools and Equipment for Simple Low-Histamine Cooking

Equipping your kitchen with the correct tools can make it easier to prepare excellent low-histamine meals. Here's a list of necessary tools and equipment that will make your culinary journey easier:

- Chef's Knife: A high-quality chef's knife is a multipurpose instrument for cutting, slicing, and dicing vegetables, fruits, and meat.
- Paring Knife: Ideal for little chores such as peeling fruits and vegetables and removing seeds.
- Cutting Board: Select a durable cutting board made of wood or plastic. Avoid bamboo since it can house bacteria.
- Mixing Bowls: A variety of mixing bowl sizes will come in helpful when preparing ingredients, marinating, or tossing salads.
- Measuring Cups and Spoons: Proper measures are essential for a successful dish.
- Pots and Pans: Purchase a few high-quality pots and pans, including a saucepan, a skillet, and a larger pot for soups and stews. Choose between

stainless steel, cast iron, and enamel-coated cookware. Avoid nonstick pans, as the coating may contain chemicals that cause histamine reactions.

- Baking Sheet: Perfect for roasting veggies, baking poultry or fish, and creating homemade granola.
- A colander is useful for draining pasta, rinsing vegetables, and washing grains.
- Whisk: Ideal for whisking eggs, preparing salads, and emulsifying sauce.
- Wooden spoons and spatulas: These will not scratch your cookware and are suitable for use with acidic ingredients.
- Tongs are useful for flipping meats and veggies while cooking.

With these tools in your kitchen, you'll be able to easily and confidently prepare tasty and healthy low-histamine meals.

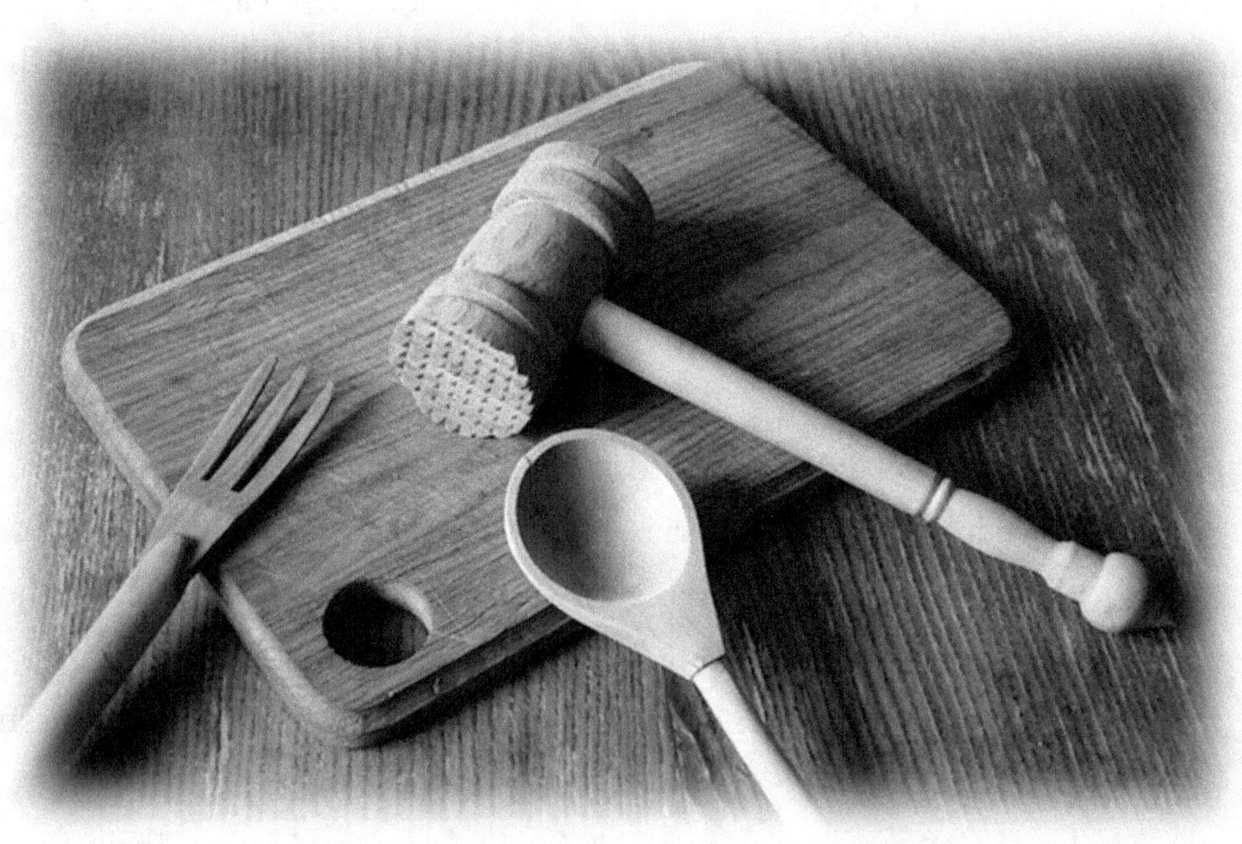

Oatmeal

Servings: Two.

Prep time: 5 minutes.

Cooking Time: 10 minutes.

Ingredients:

- One cup gluten-free rolled oats.
- 2 cups water or rice milk.
- A pinch of salt.
- Optional toppings include fresh blueberries, sliced apples, and honey.

Instructions:

- In a medium saucepan, heat the water or rice milk until it boils.
- Mix in the oats and salt.
- Reduce heat to low and cook, uncovered, for 10 minutes, stirring periodically.
- Serve hot, with optional toppings as desired.

Nutrition Information: 150 calories, 5g protein, 27g carbohydrates, 3g fat, and 4g fiber.

Oat milk Pancakes

Serves: 4

Prep time: 10 minutes.

Cook time: 15 minutes.

Ingredients:

- One cup gluten-free oat flour.
- One cup oat milk.
- One tablespoon of olive oil.
- One teaspoon of baking powder.
- A pinch of salt.

Instructions:

- In a large bowl, combine the oat flour, baking powder, and salt.
- Combine the oat milk and olive oil with the dry ingredients, stirring until just incorporated.
- Heat a nonstick pan over medium heat and lightly coat with olive oil.
- Pour 1/4 cup batter onto each pancake and heat until bubbles appear on the surface, then flip and cook until golden brown.
- Serve warm.

Nutrition Information: Calories: 120; protein: 3g; carbohydrates: 20g; fat: 3.5g.

<u>Low-Histamine Waffles</u>

Serves: 4

Prep time: 10 minutes.

Cook time: 15 minutes.

Ingredients:

- 1 cup gluten-free flour mixture.
- One cup rice milk.
- 1 tablespoon melted coconut oil.
- One teaspoon of baking powder.
- A pinch of salt.

Instructions:

- Preheat the waffle iron.
- In a mixing basin, combine the flour, baking powder, and salt.
- Mix in the rice milk and melted coconut oil until the batter is smooth.
- Pour the batter into the waffle iron and cook according to the manufacturer's directions until golden and crisp.
- Serve immediately.

Nutrition Information: 200 calories, 3g protein, 30g carbs, and 7g fat.

High-protein Blueberry Smoothie Bowl

Serves: 1

Prep time: 5 minutes.

Ingredients:

- One cup of fresh blueberries
- One-half cup rice milk
- 1/4 cup of protein powder (rice or pea protein).
- One spoonful of chia seeds.
- Ice cubes, as needed.

Instructions:

- Combine all ingredients in a blender.
- Blend on high until smooth and creamy.
- Pour into a bowl and, if preferred, top with more fresh blueberries or chia seeds.

Nutrition Information: 250 calories, 20g protein, 35g carbs, and 4g fat.

<u>**Vegan Salted Caramel Granola.**</u>

Servings: Six.

Prep time: 10 minutes.

Cook time: 20 minutes.

Ingredients:

- Two cups of gluten-free rolled oats
- 1/2 cup chopped raw almonds (as permitted)
- 1/4 cup uncooked pumpkin seeds
- One-quarter cup coconut oil
- One-quarter cup agave syrup
- One teaspoon of vanilla extract.
- One-half teaspoon sea salt

Instructions:

- Preheat the oven to 350°F (180°C), then line a baking sheet with parchment paper.
- In a large mixing bowl, add oats, almonds, and pumpkin seeds.
- In a small saucepan over low heat, combine the coconut oil, agave syrup, vanilla essence, and sea salt, stirring until thoroughly blended.
- Pour the wet components over the dry ingredients, mixing until uniformly coated.
- Spread the mixture evenly on the prepared baking sheet.
- Bake 20 minutes, stirring halfway through, or until golden brown.
- Allow the granola to cool entirely on the baking sheet; it will firm up while cooling.

Nutrition Information: 300 calories, 7g protein, 35g carbs, and 15g fat.

<u>Low-Histamine Apple Pie Smoothie</u>

Serves: 1

Prep time: 5 minutes.

Ingredients:

- One sweet apple, cored and sliced
- Half-cup frozen cauliflower florets
- Two tablespoons of gluten-free rolled oats.
- One tablespoon of macadamia nut butter.
- A little slice of fresh ginger.
- One cup rice milk.
- One tablespoon honey (optional)

Instructions:

- Combine all of the ingredients in a high-speed blender.
- Blend until smooth and creamy.
- Pour into a glass and drink immediately.

Nutrition Information: Calories: 383, protein: 19.5g, carbs: 52.9g, and fat: 12.2g.

Fluffy Vegan Green Monster Kale Pancakes

Serving size: 15 pancakes.

Prep time: 5 minutes.

Cook Time: 25 minutes.

Ingredients:

- 1-1/2 cups spelt flour
- 1/2 teaspoon baking powder.
- 1/2 teaspoon baking soda.
- 1/4 teaspoon salt.
- 3 tablespoons agave syrup.
- One cup of almond milk.
- One-third cup olive oil
- 1 teaspoon of apple cider vinegar.
- 1.5 cups of tightly packed fresh kale
- 3.5 ounces apple sauce.

Instructions:

- Combine dry ingredients in a bowl.
- Blend the wet ingredients, including the kale, until smooth.
- Combine the wet and dry ingredients.
- Cook pancakes over medium heat until browned on both sides.

Low-Histamine Blackberry Smoothie with Rainbow Chard

Serves: 1

Prep time: 5 minutes.

Ingredients:

- 100 g blackberries.
- One nectarine
- 45 grams cauliflower florets.
- 30-gram rainbow chard
- 1–2 tablespoons macadamia butter
- 200 mL rice milk

Instructions:

- Combine all ingredients in a blender.
- Blend until smooth.
- Enjoy chilled.

Mango and Moringa Smoothie Bowl

Serves: 1

Prep time: 5 minutes.

Ingredients:

- 1 cup mango (fresh or frozen)
- 1/2 cup cauliflower, frozen or lightly steamed, cooled.
- One handful of fresh moringa leaves
- 1/4–1/2 cucumber
- 1 teaspoon honey (or liquid sweetener of your choice)

Instructions:

- Combine all of the ingredients and blend until smooth.
- Transfer to a bowl and top with your favorite toppings.

<u>Homemade Muesli</u>

Servings: 4–5.

Prep time: 5 minutes.

Cook time: 7 minutes.

Ingredients:

- 1/2 cup of gluten-free rolled oats
- One handful of macadamia nuts.
- 2 tablespoons flax seeds.
- One-quarter cup pumpkin seeds
- One huge date.
- One kid-sized pack of raisins
- 1 teaspoon of olive oil.
- 2 tablespoons desiccated coconut.
- Two tablespoons of quinoa puffs.

Instructions:

- Preheat the oven to 175°C (350°F).
- Blend oats, nuts, seeds, raisins, dates, and oil till desired texture.
- Bake the mixture with coconut and quinoa puffs until the coconut browned.

<u>Ginger Sweet Potato and Carrot Soup</u>

Serves: 4

Prep time: 10 minutes.

Cook Time: 20 minutes.

Ingredients:

- Two large sweet potatoes, peeled and diced
- 4 big peeled and sliced carrots.
- One tablespoon of olive oil.
- 1 onion, chopped
- 4 cups of low histamine vegetable broth.
- 1 inch of grated fresh ginger.
- Salt to taste.

Instructions:

- Heat the olive oil in a big pot over medium heat.
- Add the onions and ginger, and sauté until transparent.
- Add the sweet potatoes and carrots and simmer for 5 minutes.
- Pour in the veggie broth and bring to a boil.
- Reduce heat to a simmer and cook for 15 minutes, or until vegetables are soft.
- Using an immersion blender, or a conventional blender in batches, blend until smooth.
- Season with salt and serve hot.

Nutrition Information: Calories: 180, protein: 3g, carbohydrates: 40g, and fat: 2g.

<u>Easy Mashed Radish</u>

Serves: 4

Prep time: 5 minutes.

Cook Time: 25 minutes.

Ingredients:

- Two bunches of radishes, trimmed and halved
- Two teaspoons of olive oil.
- Salt to taste.

Instructions:

- Cook the radishes in water until tender, about 20 minutes.
- Drain, then return to the pot.
- Add olive oil and mash until smooth.
- Season with salt and serve warm.

Nutrition Information: Calories: 70, protein: 1g, carbohydrates: 2g, and fat: 7g.

Roasted Spaghetti Squash Boats

Servings: Two.

Prep time: 10 minutes.

Cook Time: 40 minutes.

Ingredients:

- One spaghetti squash, halved and seeded
- One tablespoon of olive oil.
- Salt to taste.

Instructions:

- Preheat the oven to 400°F (200° C).
- Brush olive oil inside each squash half and season with salt.
- Place the cut side down on a baking sheet and roast for about 40 minutes, or until soft.
- With a fork, scrape out the "spaghetti" strands.
- Serve hot with your choice of low-histamine toppings.

Nutrition Information: Calories: 75, protein: 1.5g, carbohydrates: 17g, and fat: 3.5g.

<u>**Savory Sautéed Butternut Squash**</u>

Serves: 4

Prep time: 10 minutes.

Cook time: 10 minutes.

Ingredients:

- One butternut squash, peeled and cubed
- Two teaspoons of olive oil.
- Salt to taste.

Instructions:

- Heat the olive oil in a large skillet over medium heat.
- Sauté the butternut squash until golden and soft, about 10 minutes.
- Season with salt and serve warm.

Nutrition Information: Calories: 90, protein: 1g, carbs: 22g, and fat: 2g.

Microgreen Salad with Fresh Ginger Dressing.

Servings: Two.

Prep time: 5 minutes.

Ingredients:

- Two cups of assorted microgreens
- 1 grated carrot.
- 1 inch of grated fresh ginger.
- Two teaspoons of olive oil.
- One tablespoon of apple cider vinegar.
- One teaspoon of honey.
- Salt to taste.

Instructions:

- In a small container, mix together grated ginger, olive oil, apple cider vinegar, honey, and salt.
- Shake thoroughly to emulsify the dressing.
- Toss the microgreens and grated carrot in the dressing.
- Serve immediately.

Nutrition Information: Calories: 140, protein: 2g, carbohydrates: 10g, and fat: 10g.

<u>Creamy One-Pot Coconut, Ginger, And Carrot Soup</u>

Serves: 4

Prep time: 10 minutes.

Cook Time: 30 minutes.

Ingredients:

- One tablespoon of coconut oil.
- One small onion, chopped
- 2 garlic cloves, minced
- 2 tbsp fresh ginger, grated
- 1 pound peeled and diced carrots.
- One can (14 ounces) coconut milk
- 4 cups of low histamine vegetable broth.
- Salt to taste.

Instructions:

- Heat the coconut oil in a big pot over medium heat.
- Sauté the onion, garlic, and ginger until they are transparent.
- Add the carrots and simmer for 5 minutes.
- Add coconut milk and vegetable broth, and bring to a boil.
- Reduce the heat, cover, and simmer for about 25 minutes, or until the carrots are tender.
- Using an immersion blender, purée the soup until smooth.
- Season with salt and serve warm.

Nutrition Information: Calories: 250, protein: 3g, carbohydrates: 20g, and fat: 18g

Baked Crispy Turmeric Potatoes

Serves: 4

Prep time: 10 minutes.

Cook Time: 30 minutes.

Ingredients:

- 2 pounds baby potatoes, halved.
- 2 tablespoons olive oil.
- One teaspoon turmeric
- Salt to taste.

Instructions:

- Preheat the oven to 425°F (220°C).
- Toss the potatoes with olive oil, turmeric, and salt.
- Arrange on a baking sheet in a single layer.
- Bake for 30 minutes, until crispy and golden.
- Serve hot.

Nutrition Information: Calories: 200, protein: 4g, carbohydrates: 38g, and fat: 4g.

Easy Chestnut Flour Crepes.

Servings: eight crepes.

Prep time: 5 minutes.

Cook Time: 15 minutes.

Ingredients:

- One cup of chestnut flour.
- 1-1/2 cups water
- 1 egg
- One pinch of salt.
- Olive oil for cooking.

Instructions:

- Whisk together the chestnut flour, water, egg, and salt until smooth.
- Place a nonstick pan over medium heat and lightly oil.
- Pour batter to make thin crepes and heat until the edges lift.
- Turn and cook the other side until browned.
- Repeat with the remaining batter.
- Serve with the desired fillings.

Nutrition Information: Calories: 95, protein: 2g, carbohydrates: 17g, and fat: 2g.

<u>**Pomegranate Sumac Salad Dressing**</u>

Serves: 4

Prep time: 5 minutes.

Ingredients:

- 1/2 cup of pomegranate juice.
- One tablespoon olive oil.
- 1 teaspoon sumac.
- 1 teaspoon honey.
- 1/2 teaspoon grated ginger.

Instructions:

- Whisk together the pomegranate juice, olive oil, sumac, honey, and ginger until thoroughly blended.
- Taste and adjust seasoning as required.
- Drizzle over your favorite salad greens and toss until coated.
- Serve immediately.

Nutrition Information: Calories: 70, protein: 0g, carbohydrates: 8g, and fat: 4g.

<u>**Pistachio Zucchini Mint Noodles.**</u>

Serves: 4

Prep time: 10 minutes.

Cook Time: 15 minutes.

Ingredients:

- 1/4 cup unsalted pistachios.
- One garlic clove.
- 1 teaspoon thyme.
- 3/4 of a large zucchini.
- Salt to taste.
- One tablespoon olive oil.
- Fresh mint leaves.

Instructions:

- Combine pistachios, garlic, and thyme to form a coarse dust.
- In a blender, combine zucchini, salt, olive oil, and mint; pulse until smooth.
- Lightly cook the remaining zucchini slices in olive oil.
- Prepare rice noodles according to package directions and stir with sauce.
- Garnish with fresh mint leaves before serving.

Nutrition: Calories: 220, Protein: 6g, Carbohydrates: 34g, Fat: 7g.

Roasted Cauliflower

Serves: 4

Prep time: 5 minutes.

Cook Time: 20 minutes.

Ingredients:

- Cut 1 head of cauliflower into florets.
- 2 tablespoons olive oil.
- Salt to taste.

Instructions:

- Preheat the oven to 425°F.
- Toss the cauliflower with olive oil and salt.
- Roast until golden brown along the edges.
- Serve warm.

Nutritional Information: Calories: 107, Protein: 4g, Carbs: 10g, Fat: 7g

<u>**Sweet Potato Toasts.**</u>

Serves: 4

Prep time: 5 minutes.

Cook Time: 30 minutes.

Ingredients:

- Two huge sweet potatoes sliced 1/4 inch thick.
- Olive oil for brushing.

Instructions:

- Preheat the oven to 350°F.
- Coat sweet potato slices with olive oil.
- Bake until the edges are crusty.
- Serve with low-histamine toppings.

Nutritional Information: Calories: 112; protein: 2g; carbohydrates: 26g; fat: 0.1g.

<u>**Easy Herb Millet**</u>

Serves: 4

Prep time: 5 minutes.

Cook Time: 20 minutes.

Ingredients:

- One cup millet.
- Two glasses of water.
- One tablespoon olive oil.
- Fresh herbs (thyme and parsley)
- Salt to taste.

Instructions:

• Rinse the millet and boil in water until soft.

• Mix in the olive oil, fresh herbs, and salt.

• Fluff with a fork before serving.

Nutritional Information: Calories: 207, Protein: 6g, Carbs: 41g, Fat: 3.5g

<u>Pumpkin Soup</u>

Serves: 4

Prep time: 10 minutes.

Cook Time: 30 minutes.

Ingredients:

- One small pumpkin, peeled and cubed
- 1 onion, chopped
- 2 tablespoons olive oil.
- 4 cups of low histamine vegetable broth.
- Add salt and pepper to taste.

Instructions:

- Sauté the onion in olive oil until transparent.
- Add the pumpkin and simmer for a few minutes.
- Pour in the broth and bring to a boil.
- Simmer until the pumpkin is soft.
- Blend until smooth, then season with salt and pepper.
- Serve hot.

Nutritional Information: Calories: 123, Protein: 2g, Carbohydrates: 30g, Fat: 1g.

<u>**Roasted Vegetables with Tahini Sauce.**</u>

Serves: 4

Prep time: 10 minutes.

Cook Time: 30 minutes.

Ingredients:

- 8 cups of mixed vegetables, including zucchini, bell peppers, and carrots.
- 2 tablespoons olive oil.
- Salt to taste.
- 3 tablespoons tahini.
- One garlic clove, minced
- 4 tablespoons of water (add more if too thick).
- 3 1/2 tablespoons pine nuts (optional)

Instructions:

- Preheat your oven to 400°F (200°C).
- Toss the vegetables with olive oil and salt before spreading on a baking sheet.
- Roast for 30 minutes, then rotate halfway through.
- While roasting, combine the tahini, garlic, and water until smooth.
- Toast pine nuts until lightly toasted.
- Drizzle tahini sauce over the vegetables and top with pine nuts.

Nutritional Information: Calories: 300, Protein: 8g, Carbohydrates: 35g, Fat: 17g.

Carrot Risotto

Serves: 4

Prep time: 5 minutes.

Cook Time: 30 minutes.

Ingredients:

- One tablespoon olive oil.
- 1 small onion, coarsely chopped
- 1 cup arborio rice.
- Three cups of low histamine vegetable broth.
- 2 big carrots pureed
- Salt to taste.

Instructions:

- Heat olive oil in a pan and sauté the onion until transparent.
- Add rice and simmer for 2 minutes.
- Gradually add the broth and mix until absorbed.
- Stir in the pureed carrots and simmer until creamy.
- Season with salt and serve warm

Nutritional Information: Calories: 210, Protein: 4g, Carbohydrates: 40g, Fat: 3g.

<u>**Sweet Potato Waffles.**</u>

Serves: 4

Prep time: 10 minutes.

Cook Time: 15 minutes.

Ingredients: 7

- One large sweet potato, boiled and mashed
- 2 eggs
- One-half cup rice milk
- One cup gluten-free flour.
- One teaspoon of baking powder.
- A pinch of salt.

Instructions:

- Preheat the waffle iron.
- Combine mashed sweet potatoes, eggs, and rice milk.
- Combine flour, baking powder, and salt; stir until smooth.
- Pour batter into the waffle iron and cook until golden.
- Serve with tolerated toppings

Nutritional Information: Calories: 220, Protein: 6g, Carbohydrates: 40g, Fat: 4g.

<u>**Rice Cakes With Shmear**</u>

Servings: Two.

Prep time: 5 minutes.

Ingredients:

- Two ordinary rice cakes.
- 2 tablespoons macadamia nut butter or sunflower butter.
- Optional toppings include mashed blueberries and thinly sliced apples.

Instructions:

- Spread 1 tablespoon macadamia or sunflower butter on each rice cake.
- Add optional toppings if desired.
- Serve immediately.

Nutritional information: 180 calories, 3g protein, 20g carbs, and 10g fat.

<u>**Sweetened Low Histamine Fruits**</u>

Serves: 4

Prep time: 10 minutes.

Ingredients:

- One cup blueberry.
- One apple, diced
- One pear, diced
- Optional: sprinkle with honey or coconut cream.

Instructions:

- In a serving bowl, combine blueberries, apples, and pears.
- Drizzle with honey or coconut cream if desired.
- Serve fresh.

Nutritional information: 95 calories, 1g protein, 25g carbs, and 0.5g fat.

Carrot Sticks with Low Histamine Ranch.

Serves: 4

Prep time: 10 minutes.

Ingredients:

- 4 large carrots peeled and sliced into sticks.
- For ranch dressing:
- 1/2 cup of coconut yogurt.
- One tablespoon olive oil.
- 1 teaspoon of apple cider vinegar (optional)
- Fresh herbs (parsley, dill), finely chopped.
- Salt to taste.

Instructions:

- In a small mixing bowl, combine coconut yogurt, olive oil, apple cider vinegar (if using), and fresh herbs.
- Season with salt to taste.
- Serve carrot sticks with ranch dressing for dipping.

Nutritional information: 70 calories, 1g protein, 8g carbs, and 4g fat.

<u>**Butternut Squash Hummus**</u>

Serves: 4

Prep time: 10 minutes.

Cook Time: 30 minutes.

Ingredients:

- 250-gram butternut squash, roasted and mashed
- One-quarter cup basil leaves
- 1/2 cup macadamia nuts.
- 2 tablespoons olive oil.
- 1 teaspoon cumin.
- 1/4 teaspoon sea salt.
- Optional: 1/2 teaspoon of apple cider vinegar or lemon juice.

Instructions:

- Preheat the oven to 340°F (170° C). Roast the butternut squash till soft.
- In a food processor, combine basil leaves to make a paste.
- Add the macadamia nuts and olive oil, and blend until smooth.
- Mix in the roasted squash, cumin, salt, and apple cider vinegar or lemon juice, if using. Blend until completely combined.
- Serve as a dip or spread.

Nutritional Information: Calories: 226; protein: 2g; carbohydrates: 20g; fat: 16g.

Ginger Carrot and Apple Muffins

Servings: 12 muffins.

Prep time: 20 minutes.

Cook Time: 35 minutes.

Ingredients:

- 1/2 cup rice or oat milk.
- One tablespoon of lemon juice or apple cider vinegar.
- Two medium-sized carrots, shredded
- One medium apple, shredded
- 1 cup chopped macadamia nuts.
- One and one-third cups buckwheat flour
- One tablespoon of ground flaxseed.
- Two tablespoons tapioca flour
- One tablespoon of ground ginger
- 1 teaspoon baking powder (gluten-free).
- 1/2 teaspoon bicarbonate soda
- 1/4 teaspoon salt.
- 3 eggs
- 3 tbsp and 1 tsp olive oil
- 4 tablespoons honey.

Instructions:

- Preheat the oven to 356°F (180°C) and line a muffin tin with paper liners.
- Combine rice milk with ACV to make 'buttermilk'. Set aside.
- Mix together buckwheat flour, flaxseed, tapioca flour, bicarb, baking powder, salt, and ginger.

- In another bowl, combine the eggs, olive oil, honey, and 'buttermilk'.
- Combine wet and dry ingredients, then mix in carrots, apples, and nuts.
- Divide the batter among the muffin cups and bake until firm and brown.
- Keep in an airtight container or freeze.

Nutritional Information: Calories: 222, Protein: 4g, Carbs: 33g, Fat: 9g

<u>Roasted Zucchini Dip</u>

Servings: Six.

Prep time: 5 minutes.

Cook Time: 15 minutes.

Ingredients:

- Five zucchinis.
- Three cloves of garlic.
- One-third cup extra virgin olive oil
- One cup basil or coriander leaves.
- One teaspoon of sea salt.
- 1/4 tsp black or white pepper.

Instructions:

- Preheat the oven to 200C (390F).
- Peel the zucchini and cut off the top and bottom.
- Cut zucchini into ½ inch thick strips, drizzle with olive oil, and set in a roasting pan with whole garlic cloves.
- Roast until tender (around 15 minutes).
- In a food processor or blender, mix together the roasted zucchini, olive oil, garlic, basil leaves, and salt.
- Pulse until thick purée.
- Serve warm or keep in the fridge

Nutritional Information: Calories: 136kcal, Carbohydrates: 6g, Protein: 2g, Fat: 13g, Fiber: 2g

Apple Spiced Oatmeal Cookies

Serving size: 12 cookies.

Prep time: 10 minutes.

Cook Time: 15 minutes.

Ingredients:

- One cup gluten-free flour.
- 1.5 cups oats (rolled is ideal)
- 2 teaspoons baking powder.
- One teaspoon of ground ginger
- 1/4 teaspoon sea salt.
- 1/4 cup macadamia nuts, chopped
- Two tablespoons of ground flax seed
- One egg or chia egg.
- One-half cup coconut sugar
- 1/2 cup coconut oil, melted
- 1 apple, coarsely chopped.

Instructions:

- Preheat the oven to 180C (350F) and line a baking sheet with parchment paper.
- In a large mixing bowl, add flour, oats, baking powder, ginger, sea salt, and macadamia nuts.
- In a separate bowl, combine the ground flax, egg, coconut sugar, melted coconut oil, and diced apple.
- Combine the wet and dry ingredients to make a dough.

- Using a 1/4 cup, spoon balls of dough onto the baking sheet and lightly press down.
- Bake for 15 minutes and cool before serving

Nutritional Information: Calories: 277kcal, Carbohydrates: 27g, Protein: 3g, Fat: 13g

Homemade French Fries

Serves: 4

Prep time: 10 minutes.

Cook Time: 30 minutes.

Ingredients:

- Baked potatoes
- lard or high heat-safe fat (refined avocado oil, refined coconut oil, tallow, ghee, or butter).
- Dried rosemary and garlic (optional).

Instructions:

- Wash potatoes and cut into fries.
- Toss in fat and optional seasonings.
- Cook at 450°F (230°C) until crispy

Sweet Potatoes

Serves: 4

Prep time: 5 minutes.

Cook Time: 30 minutes.

Ingredients:

- Sweet Potatoes
- Olive Oil.
- Salt

Instructions:

- Preheat the oven to 400°F (205° C).
- Wash and slice the sweet potatoes.
- Place on a baking pan, drizzle with oil and season with salt.
- Roast until tender.

Vegetables With Low Histamine Salad Dressings

Ingredients:

- Your choice of low histamine vegetables.
- Olive Oil.
- Herbs and spices, as tolerated.

Instructions:

- Prepare your desired vegetables.
- Combine olive oil, herbs, and spices to make a dressing.
- Toss vegetables with dressing and serve.

Pistachio Nigella Halva.

Servings: eight.

Prep time: 5 minutes.

Freeze for 3 hours.

Ingredients:

- 85 g pistachios.
- One-half cup maple syrup
- One cup light tahini.

Instructions:

- Heat the oven to 180°C. Roast the pistachios for about 8 minutes, or until golden.
- In a saucepan, bring maple syrup to a boil and allow to bubble for 2-3 minutes.
- Remove from heat and whisk in the tahini until smooth and firm.
- Stir in the chopped pistachios.
- Line a small baking tray with parchment paper and evenly distribute the ingredients.
- To set, freeze for about 3 hours. Then chop and serve.

Nutritional Information: Calories: 300, Protein: 8g, Carbs: 18g, Fat: 23g

Candied Nut or Seed

Serves: 4

Prep time: 5 minutes.

Cook Time: 20 minutes.

Ingredients:

- 1 cup nuts or seeds of your choice.
- 2 tsp low histamine sweetener (such as maple syrup)
- One pinch of salt.

Instructions:

- Preheat the oven to 350°F (175° C).
- In a bowl, combine nuts or seeds, sweetener, and salt.
- Place on a baking sheet and bake until toasted

Nutritional information: calories: 180, protein: 5g, carbohydrates: 8g, fat: 16g.

<u>Creamy Vegan Fruit Dip.</u>

Servings: eight.

Prep time: 5 minutes.

Ingredients:

- One-half cup almond butter
- One-half cup coconut cream
- One tablespoon maple syrup.
- 1/2 teaspoon vanilla powder.

Instructions:

- In a mixing bowl, combine almond butter, coconut cream, maple syrup, and vanilla powder until smooth.
- Serve alongside fresh fruit slices

Nutritional Information: Calories: 150, Protein: 4g, Carbs: 7g, Fat: 13g

Easy Homemade Peppermint Syrup

Serves: 16

Prep time: 5 minutes.

Cook Time: 5 minutes.

Ingredients:

- One cup of water.
- 1 cup low histamine sweetener (such as allulose)
- 1 teaspoon of peppermint extract.

Instructions:

- In a saucepan, heat water and sweetener until dissolved.
- Remove from the heat and add the peppermint extract.
- Let cool before using

Nutritional Information: Calories: 50, Protein: 0g, Carbohydrates: 13g, and Fat: 0g.

<u>**Easy Saffron Syrup**</u>

Serves: 16

Prep time: 5 minutes.

Cook Time: 5 minutes.

Ingredients:

- One cup of water.
- 1 cup low histamine sweetener (such as allulose)
- 1 pinch of saffron threads

Instructions:

- In a saucepan, combine all of the ingredients and heat until boiling.
- Reduce the heat and simmer until the sugar dissolves and the syrup is infused with saffron.
- Allow to cool until room temperature

Nutritional Information: Calories: 50, Protein: 0g, Carbohydrates: 13g, and Fat: 0g.

<u>**Easy Cardamom Simple Syrup**</u>

Serves: 16

Prep time: 5 minutes.

Cook Time: 15 minutes.

Ingredients:

- One cup of water.
- One cup of granulated sweetener (allulose or monk fruit blend).
- 1 tablespoon cardamom seeds, finely ground

Instructions:

- Optional: Toast cardamom seeds over low heat for 3-5 minutes.
- In a saucepan, heat water until it simmers.
- Add the sweetener, stir until dissolved, and heat to a low boil.
- Add the cardamom seeds and cook on low for 10 minutes, stirring regularly.
- Remove from heat and let alone for 15-20 minutes to infuse.
- Strain and place in an airtight container.

Nutritional Information: Calories: 50, Protein: 0g, Carbohydrates: 13g, and Fat: 0g.

Easy Candied Macadamia Nut Recipe

Serves: 4

Prep time: 5 minutes.

Cook time: 10 minutes.

Ingredients:

- One cup raw macadamia nut.
- 1.5 teaspoons of low histamine sweetener (tapioca syrup or honey).
- One pinch of salt.

Instructions:

- Preheat the oven to 285°F.
- In a bowl, sprinkle syrup or honey over the nuts.
- Toss the sweetener mixture and salt to coat.
- Bake until caramelized.

Nutrition Information: Calories: 204, Protein: 2g, Carbohydrates: 4g, Fat: 21g.

Easy Chia and Flax Seed Pudding

Servings: Two.

Prep time: 5 minutes.

Ingredients:

- 1 cup non-dairy milk (macadamia, coconut)
- 2 tablespoons chia seeds.
- 2 tablespoons flaxseed meal.
- One teaspoon of vanilla powder.
- A sweetener to taste (honey or maple syrup)

Instructions:

- In a mixing bowl, combine all of the ingredients and stir for about a minute.
- Transfer to a glass container and refrigerate for an hour or more to set

Nutritional Information: Calories: 150, Protein: 4g, Carbs: 13g, Fat: 9g.

<u>Vanilla Coconut Flaxseed Pudding</u>

Servings: Two.

Prep time: 5 minutes.

Ingredients:

- 1 cup non-dairy milk (macadamia, coconut)
- 2 tablespoons flaxseed meal.
- A sweetener to taste (honey or maple syrup)
- One teaspoon of vanilla powder.
- Optional: Coconut chips.

Instructions:

- Combine milk, flax meal, sweetener, vanilla powder, and coconut chips (if using) in a mixing dish.
- Pour into a container and refrigerate for at least an hour to set.

Nutritional Information: Calories: 150, Protein: 3g, Carbs: 11g, Fat: 11g.

<u>28-Day Meal Plan</u>

Week 1:

Day 1:

- Breakfast: oatmeal.
- Lunch: Ginger Sweet Potato Carrot Soup.
- Dinner: Pistachio, zucchini, and mint noodles.
- Snack: Rice Cakes and Shmear
- Dessert: Pistachio Nigella Halva.

Day 2:

- Breakfast: High-protein blueberry smoothie bowl.
- Lunch: Easy Mashed Radish.
- Dinner: Roasted cauliflower.
- Snack: Sweetened low histamine fruits
- Dessert: candied nuts or seeds.

Day 3:

- Breakfast: vegan salted caramel granola.
- Lunch: Roasted spaghetti squash boats.
- Dinner: Sweet potato toasts.
- Snack: carrot sticks with low histamine ranch.
- Dessert: Creamy Vegan Fruit dip.

Day 4:

- Breakfast: Low Histamine Apple Pie Smoothie.

- Lunch: Savory sautéed butternut squash.

- Dinner: Easy Herbed Millet

- Snack: Butternut squash hummus.

- Dessert: Easy Homemade Peppermint Syrup

Day 5:

- Breakfast: Fluffy Vegan Green Monster Kale Pancakes.

- Lunch: Microgreen salad with fresh ginger dressing.

- Dinner: Pumpkin soup.

- Snack: Ginger-Carrot and Apple Muffins

- Dessert: Easy Saffron Syrup

Day 6:

- Breakfast: low histamine blackberry smoothie with rainbow chard

- Lunch: Creamy one-pot coconut ginger carrot soup.

- Dinner: Roasted vegetables with tahini sauce.

- Snack: Roasted zucchini dip.

- Dessert: Easy Cardamom Simple Syrup

Day 7:

- Breakfast: A Mango and Moringa Smoothie bowl.

- Lunch: Baked Crispy Turmeric Potatoes

- Dinner: carrot risotto.

- Snack: Apple Spiced Oatmeal Cookies.

- Dessert: Easy Candied Macadamia Nut Recipe

Week 2:

Day 8:

- Breakfast: oatmeal.
- Lunch: Ginger Sweet Potato Carrot Soup.
- Dinner: Pistachio, zucchini, and mint noodles.
- Snack: Rice Cakes and Shmear
- Dessert: Pistachio Nigella Halva.

Day 9:

- Breakfast: High-protein blueberry smoothie bowl.
- Lunch: Easy Mashed Radish.
- Dinner: Roasted cauliflower.
- Snack: Sweetened low histamine fruits
- Dessert: candied nuts or seeds.

Day 10:

- Breakfast: vegan salted caramel granola.
- Lunch: Roasted spaghetti squash boats.
- Dinner: Sweet potato toasts.
- Snack: carrot sticks with low histamine ranch.
- Dessert: creamy vegan fruit dip.

Day 11:

- Breakfast: Low Histamine Apple Pie Smoothie.
- Lunch: Savory sautéed butternut squash.
- Dinner: Easy Herbed Millet
- Snack: Butternut squash hummus.
- Dessert: Easy Homemade Peppermint Syrup

Day 12:

- Breakfast: Fluffy Vegan Green Monster Kale Pancakes.
- Lunch: Microgreen salad with fresh ginger dressing.
- Dinner: Pumpkin soup.
- Snack: Ginger-Carrot and Apple Muffins
- Dessert: Easy Saffron Syrup

Day 13:

- Breakfast: low histamine blackberry smoothie with rainbow chard
- Lunch: Creamy one-pot coconut ginger carrot soup.
- Dinner: Roasted vegetables with tahini sauce.
- Snack: Roasted zucchini dip.
- Dessert: Easy Cardamom Simple Syrup

Day 14:

- Breakfast: a mango and moringa smoothie bowl.
- Lunch: Baked Crispy Turmeric Potatoes
- Dinner: carrot risotto.
- Snack: Apple Spiced Oatmeal Cookies.
- Dessert: Easy Candied Macadamia Nut Recipe

Week 3:

Day 15:

- Breakfast: homemade muesli.
- Lunch: Pomegranate Sumac Salad Dressing with Mixed Greens.
- Dinner: Sweet potato waffles.
- Snack: Homemade French fries.
- Dessert: Easy Chia and Flax Seed Pudding

Day 16:

- Breakfast: Oat milk Pancakes
- Lunch is Ginger Sweet Potato Carrot Soup.
- Dinner: Roasted vegetables with tahini sauce.
- Snack: Sweet potatoes.
- Dessert: Vanilla Coconut Flax Seed Pudding.

Day 17:

- Breakfast: low histamine waffles
- Lunch: Easy Chestnut Flour Crepes
- Dinner: carrot risotto.
- Snack: Vegetables with low histamine salad dressing.
- Dessert: Pistachio Nigella Halva.

Day 18:

- Breakfast: High-protein blueberry smoothie bowl.
- Lunch: Easy Mashed Radish.
- Dinner: Roasted cauliflower.
- Snack: Rice Cakes and Shmear
- Dessert: candied nuts or seeds.

Day 19:

- Breakfast: vegan salted caramel granola.
- Lunch: Roasted spaghetti squash boats.
- Dinner: Sweet potato toasts.
- Snack: Sweetened low histamine fruits
- Dessert: creamy vegan fruit dip.

Day 20:

- Breakfast: Low Histamine Apple Pie Smoothie.
- Lunch: Savory sautéed butternut squash.
- Dinner: Easy Herbed Millet
- Snack: carrot sticks with low histamine ranch.
- Dessert: Easy Homemade Peppermint Syrup

Day 21:

- Breakfast: Fluffy Vegan Green Monster Kale Pancakes.
- Lunch: Microgreen salad with fresh ginger dressing.
- Dinner: Pumpkin soup.
- Snack: Butternut squash hummus.
- Dessert: Easy Saffron Syrup

Week 4:

Day 22:

- Breakfast: Oat milk Pancakes
- Lunch: Pomegranate Sumac Salad Dressing with Mixed Greens.
- Dinner: Sweet potato waffles.
- Snack: Homemade French fries.
- Dessert: Easy Chia and Flax Seed Pudding

Day 23:

- Breakfast: low histamine waffles
- Lunch: Ginger Sweet Potato Carrot Soup.
- Dinner: Roasted vegetables with tahini sauce.
- Snack: Sweet potatoes.
- Dessert: Vanilla Coconut Flax Seed Pudding.

Day 24:

- Breakfast: High-protein blueberry smoothie bowl.
- Lunch: Easy Mashed Radish.
- Dinner: Roasted cauliflower.
- Snack: Rice Cakes and Shmear
- Dessert: candied nuts or seeds.

Day 25:

- Breakfast: vegan salted caramel granola.
- Lunch: Roasted spaghetti squash boats.
- Dinner: Sweet potato toasts.
- Snack: Sweetened low histamine fruits
- Dessert: creamy vegan fruit dip.

Day 26:

- Breakfast: Low Histamine Apple Pie Smoothie.
- Lunch: Savory sautéed butternut squash.
- Dinner: Easy Herbed Millet
- Snack: carrot sticks with low histamine ranch.
- Dessert: Easy Homemade Peppermint Syrup

Day 27:

- Breakfast: Fluffy Vegan Green Monster Kale Pancakes.
- Lunch: Microgreen salad with fresh ginger dressing.
- Dinner: Pumpkin soup.
- Snack: Butternut squash hummus.
- Dessert: Easy Saffron Syrup

Day 28:

- Breakfast: low histamine blackberry smoothie with rainbow chard
- Lunch: Creamy one-pot coconut ginger carrot soup.
- Dinner: Roasted vegetables with tahini sauce.
- Snack: Roasted zucchini dip.
- Dessert: Easy Cardamom Simple Syrup

<u>**Tips for Dining Out**</u>

Dining out while on a low histamine diet might be difficult, but with careful planning and communication, you can still enjoy a meal at a restaurant. Here are some ideas to help you eat out safely:

- **Research the Restaurant**: Before going out, check the restaurant's menu online to see if there are any low-histamine options available. You can also phone ahead to see whether they can meet your dietary needs.

- **Speak with the staff**: When you arrive, tell the waiter or chef about your dietary limitations. Explain what histamine intolerance is and which foods you should avoid.

- **Avoid Certain Foods:** Aged, fermented, and processed foods are often rich in histamine. This includes aged cheeses, wine, smoked meats, and some fish.

- **Bring Your Own Snacks**: If you're worried about the menu options, bring some low-histamine snacks as a backup.

- **Choose Simple Dishes:** Recipes with fewer ingredients are less likely to contain hidden histamines. Grilled meats and cooked veggies are often safe choices.

- **Ask for Substitutions**: Do not be afraid to request substitutions. Request fresh herbs instead of spice blends, or olive oil and vinegar instead of ready-made dressings.

- **Carry a Histamine List**: Use a list of high-histamine meals as a reference when ordering.

- **Don't Forget Your medicine**: If you've been prescribed medicine for histamine sensitivity, keep it with you in case of inadvertent exposure1.

- **Do Something Calming**: Stress can worsen histamine intolerance symptoms, so try to unwind before and throughout your meal3.
- **Reframe Your Thoughts**: Rather of focusing on the limits, consider dining out as an opportunity to sample new, safe meals while also enjoying the social experience.

Remember that good communication is essential, and don't be hesitant to ask for what you need. Most restaurants are willing to accommodate dietary restrictions to ensure that their clients enjoy a positive eating experience.

Managing Symptoms and Flare-ups

Managing symptoms and flare-ups associated with histamine intolerance requires a combination of dietary changes, lifestyle changes, and possibly medication. Here are some techniques for managing symptoms:

- **Identify and Avoid Triggers**: Keep a detailed food journal to chronicle your eating habits and any symptoms that arise. This might help you discover and avoid foods that cause symptoms.
- **Dietary Management**: Eat a low-histamine diet and avoid high-histamine items such aged cheeses, cured meats, fermented foods, and alcohol. Instead, focus on fresh, unadulterated food.
- **Medication**: If prescribed by a healthcare physician, drugs such as antihistamines can help alleviate symptoms. Always have your medication with you in case of inadvertent exposure.
- **Stress Management**: Stress can increase symptoms, so incorporate stress-relieving activities into your daily routine, such as meditation, yoga, or deep breathing.

- **Cold Therapy:** Putting an ice pack on your head or back can help calm the body's reaction by lowering blood vessel dilatation and the sense of heat.
- **Modify Your Diet**: Based on your observations from the food diary, change the quantity and frequency of particular foods to maintain a healthy balance.
- **Consult a dietician:** Create a specific food plan with the help of a dietician who understands histamine intolerance.
- **Cook at Home:** Preparing your own meals allows you to manage the ingredients and guarantees that the food is fresh and low in histamine.
- **Supplements**: Some people may benefit from taking vitamin C and quercetin, which can help stabilize mast cells and minimize histamine release. Before using any supplements, consult with a healthcare practitioner.
- **Stay Informed**: Stay up to date on the latest research and suggestions for treating histamine intolerance.

CONCLUSION

As we come to the end of this culinary journey, I hope "The Low Histamine Cookbook" has presented you with not only a selection of tasty dishes, but also a roadmap to navigating your diet confidently and creatively. Each dish was carefully developed, keeping in mind the balance and variety required to make every meal both safe and enjoyable.

Your health and well-being have been at the forefront of this work, and it is my honest hope that this cookbook will become a treasured tool in your kitchen, assisting you in managing histamine intolerance and enjoying food to its full potential.

If you enjoyed and valued these recipes, I would appreciate it if you could give some positive feedback or an honest review. Your views and experiences are essential, not just to me, but also to others on similar nutritional paths. Sharing your opinions can help to build a community of support and information, which is critical for all of us on this path.

Thank you for making this cookbook a part of your culinary journey. May your meals be enjoyable, your symptoms manageable, and your days full with the simple pleasures of delicious cuisine.